SARDINE SOLUTION

HOW AND WHY TO EAT THE WORLD'S MOST BADASS SOURCE OF PROTEIN

K. SUZANNE

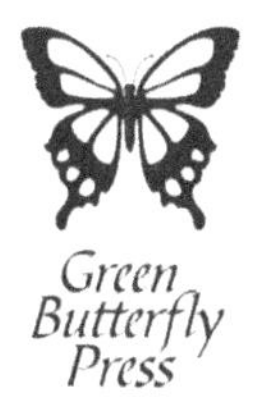

Green
Butterfly
Press

ABOUT THE AUTHOR

Kristen Suzanne is an author traveling the world with her family on a multi-year odyssey to experience other cultures and stay fit while she stuffs her face with their food. (For now, meat anyway.)

Kristen's blog at: **GlobalKristen.com**

Twitter: @KristensRaw

Instagram: global_kristen

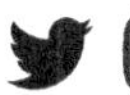

CONTENTS

INTRODUCTION

For a free, printable .PDF of the recipes in this book, email me at kristen@globalkristen.com.

My 7-year old humored me as she pulled the spine out of the sardine, gleefully exclaiming in her best Gollum voice, "I must eat the spine!" She tipped her head back, mouth wide open, dangled the wiggly spine over her mouth, and dropped it in. The sardine spine-drop has become one of her regular party tricks these days. It never fails to mesmerize the other kids.

Sardines are not super popular, even among people who seek good sources of protein for health and fitness reasons. This book aims to change that. Many people love the taste of sardines, but many others do not, claiming they taste too fishy. This latter group either aren't preparing the fish properly, or in the case of recipes that don't mute the strong flavor, they haven't yet acquired the taste. Or they're not having enough fun with sardines, like my daughter does.

Regardless, everyone should eat more sardines. They're an absolute superfood. Sardines are glorious and superior. They're nutritious and cheap. They're also extremely tasty, if you prepare them correctly. Sardines are one of my favorite foods, period. It's amazing that one food can tick so many boxes: nutritious, convenient, dirt cheap – all in one cool little pocket-sized metal box. They taste great, too, once you learn what to do with these little pieces of natural perfection from the sea. You can even eat them any time of day, as an excellent breakfast, lunch, dinner, or snack.

As a person who gets excited about superfoods, I was initially drawn to sardines by their insanely good nutrition. So, if you need a gentle nudge (or a shove) to consider sardines as one of your go-to sources of protein, think about this:

- Sardines are 78% protein (good for strength building, increased performance, weight loss and maintenance)
- They're high in omega-3 fatty acids, which decrease inflammation (vital for your brain health, cardiovascular system, and metabolism)
- They contain B vitamins along with vitamin D, CoQ10, calcium, potassium, phosphorous, and more (important for your teeth, skin, heart, and energy levels).
- They're very LOW in mercury, a neurotoxic heavy metal. (More on this later.) This is in contrast to other meaty fish that are higher on the food chain, like tuna. If you eat fish (and you should), then you can't do better than the humble sardine.

My Sardine Story

My first experience with sardines was not until my twenties, when my stepdad ate them. I had never tried them. I thought the whole idea was gross. The look and smell were enough to put me off. But he loved them. He was always trying too convince me that, "No, they're not cat food."

Oh, but things change.

Twenty years later, when my family stopped eating a vegan diet (because our health was deteriorating), sardines were one of the first animal foods I introduced. We wanted to eat fish, and in our research, sardines kept coming up at the top of the list, due to their superior nutrition and low trophic level (i.e., the position on the food chain). Sardines were routinely labeled as a "superfood" in the paleo food community. That turned me on. Thus began my grand sardine adventure.

I nervously bought two cans. I brought them home. I steeled myself by studying the box details about all of the nutrients I was about to eat. I called my family into the kitchen... this was a big deal. I opened the box, then the can. I looked at the little silver headless fish. I got scared. I gave the fork and can to Greg, my husband. He took the can, forked a sardine, put it in his mouth whole. He chewed and swallowed. He said they were actually pretty good. (Okay, he had eaten loads of sardines as a kid, with ketchup, on Saltine crackers.)

I was inspired again. After I watched him eat one, I tried it myself, but I covered mine in mustard, lemon juice and sauerkraut. And? I was surprised to realize that, no, it wasn't bad.

But I definitely wasn't in love. The flavor was fine, actually. For me, the difficult parts were the texture and look, because I could see and feel the tiny bones. It's okay to eat the bones; it's just the spine, a tad gritty, not the throat-stabby-needle type of fish bones that kill you. I knew that sardines are super healthy for you, bones and all, but I was not enjoying that aspect of the experience, and the first few times I ate them, the bones skeeved me out a bit.

Some people liken smoked sardines to tuna fish. As a kid, I used to love tuna fish, but sardines were a whole new ball of wax, coming with skin, bones and all. Funny though, I have to agree... once you mash them up, it turns out sardines aren't that different from a plain ol' can of tuna.

I was determined to have more sardines in my life, but I needed to make some changes to overcome the aspects I didn't like. So I came up with a bunch of recipes to help me love them. The simplest of those recipes are contained in this book (and the rest are in my other book, "Recipes with Sardines").

For starters – and this was a real breakthrough for me – when you purée the ingredients, you can't tell the bones are in it. (You can buy boneless, skinless sardines, but I prefer them with bones for the superior nutrition.)

Over time, as I became more accustomed to the sardines' flavor by eating them multiple times a week, I soon found myself genuinely liking them, eventually craving them. At that point, I even began to enjoy eating the fish straight out of the can, no food processing or strong flavors added to mask the fish's natural texture and flavor.

Today, I'm a genuine fan of sardines and consider myself a pro at eating them. Most times, I just eat them straight from the can. With repeated exposure and some good recipes for variety, it wasn't long before they became a regular part of my diet. I guess it's true for both kids and adults... expose yourself enough times and you'll end up liking something. (Now, if I could only do that with liver. Still working on that.)

For people who aren't familiar with sardines or who might have an aversion to them, sardines are actually fun because you can vary the recipe based on whatever you have on hand. When I'm in a creative mood, I add caramelized onions. Or I add fresh green onion and celery. Sometimes, I purée sardines with roasted red bell pepper and butter... absolutely delicious. Fresh herbs are also dynamite sardine companions, and so is roasted garlic, or even avocado.

And that's just the diversity with recipes. You also have plenty of choices just buying them in the store. Canned sardines come in a variety of flavors and options. The canned fish section of your local grocery store will usually have at least one or two varieties of canned sardines. Good stores will have many varieties. You can find canned sardines packed in spring water or a wide variety of oils, sauces, herbs, etc. They're usually smoked, but on occasion they're not. We prefer the smoked variety but we'll happily eat them all. And, as mentioned before, you'll see some cans have the sardines including skin & bones and the others that are skinless & boneless.

The choice is up to you for which "flavor" of sardines you use. Have fun and try them all, with bones and without, too. This book will get you started with some carefully selected, beginner recipes. Their explicit goal (and the goal of this book), is to take you from wherever you are today on the sardine-eating spectrum, and level you up to Sardine Badass, meaning you have no problem (or even enjoy) eating sardines straight from the can. Because at that point, it becomes very easy to consume sardines in large quantities (even daily), which is where their nutrition, convenience, and even financial (low-cost) benefits can really become a cumulative, legitimately life-changing upgrade. This is what I call the "Sardine Solution." It culminates with sardines as one of your primary staples and perhaps even your biggest source of protein.

If you'd like more ways to get sardines into your diet (or make them more appealing to your less enthusiastic family members), see my other book, "Recipes with Sardines," which is a more general audience recipe book and not designed to convert sardine-haters into Sardine Badasses, but rather, to give anybody more ways to experiment with and enjoy these wonderful little fishies.

For now though, the book you're currently reading is all you need to get on the path to enjoying sardines with some fun recipes, and eventually become happy to eat them from a can straight. Plain and badass!

ONE

SARDINES BASICS

Canned sardines have become more popular in recent years, as people realize what an amazingly cool and convenient source of protein they are. They make meal prep a snap and are a fast and fun way to eat more fish without stinking up the house from cooking.

Sardines require no refrigeration and have a shelf-life of up to *five years*. And after five years, they may still be safe to eat, albeit with degraded flavor.

This makes sardines great for travel (camping, road trips, airports), and a can easily fits in a backpack or purse. In a nutshell, sardines are a delicious, easy-to-use "protein in a can." They are a mom's dream food. I can whip them into an easy meal and I can use them to stay fit and healthy.

About Sardines

Sardines are named after the lovely Italian island of Sardinia, where they were historically abundant. Sardines are small, saltwater, oily-rich, soft-boned, silvery fishes. In fact, the word "sardines" is a common name describing the immature fish of a variety of species all around the world. Portugal is one of the leading sardine-producing countries, though you can easily find varieties of them in the Atlantic Ocean, Pacific Ocean, and the Mediterranean Sea. So when you say "sardine," you are actually referring to several species of fish.

Some people seem to have a sort of psychological resistance preventing them from even trying sardines, let alone making them a regular part of their daily diet. It's time to stop that madness, as sardines are one of the most accessible superfoods in existence.

Types of Sardines You Can Buy

There are many flavors and options when it comes to eating canned sardines. (Fresh sardines are also available at some stores, but in this book, we're referring to the canned variety for their extreme convenience as part of a total "Sardine Solution.") Sardines' flesh is rich, dense, and oily and they're a nutrition powerhouse. Typically, at the cannery, the fish are washed and the heads removed. Then, the fish are smoked or cooked, and dried, packed in water/sauce/oil, and canned.

When shopping for sardines, you can opt for sardines *with skin and bones* or go *without skin and bones* ("skinless/boneless"). Some sardines are canned whole, but (thankfully) most have their heads, gills, and scales removed. If you want to avoid bones, look for them sold as "fillets." However, the bones give these little fish an extra nutrition boost of calcium, so don't be shy. The bones are fun (and quick) to chew up once you get used to it and embrace sardines as one of your favorite foods. When puréed into a pâté, you'll never even know they're there.

Next, you can choose what the sardines are packed in. Common options include:

- Water
- Olive oil (or other vegetable oils)
- Spicy chili
- Lemon
- Marinara or tomato sauce
- No salt added
- Mustard
- Hot sauce
- … and more.

Depending on where you are in the world, you'll see great variety in what sardines are packed in. As a digital nomad family moving around the world, we've found even more flavors and options on our journey, which is exciting. I like them all, except those packed in sunflower, canola, or soybean oils, which are highly inflammatory (but that's a topic for another book). Suffice it to say, the amount of any oils in a can is pretty small and you can always drain it. Still, I prefer olive oil for health, taste, and texture.

As mentioned, you'll likely find a selection at your local grocery store. It's also fun to investigate delis and Italian specialty foods stores. Once you find a brand and flavors you like, head to Amazon.com, which has a nice selection. Order using their "Subscribe and Save" feature, where you'll save money buying in bulk. Also consider checking out your local bulk-buying store like Costco or Sam's Club.

A note on size: For those new to sardines who seek the most mild taste, the rule-of-thumb says that the smaller the sardine, the milder the flavor. I agree. The bones are also smaller. And the fish fit better on a cracker whole when they're small. But sometimes I get a can that has fatter sardines in them. I either make them into pâté or give them to my aquatic hunter-gatherer husband.

Low Toxicity

Sardines, by definition, are small (young pilchards) and they are near the bottom of the aquatic food chain because they feed solely on plankton. For both of these reasons, they do not concentrate mercury or other heavy metals and PCBs that accumulate in the fatty tissue of larger and carnivorous fish, such as tuna and salmon. This means that you can consume multiple servings of sardines every day without worrying about consuming these toxins.

FAQ

How long do canned sardines last once opened and stored in the refrigerator?

Once opened, canned sardines can last for 3 to 4 days in the refrigerator. If you're saving some after opening the can, it's optimal to transfer them to a sealed glass or plastic container.

Can you freeze canned sardines?

Yes, canned sardines can be frozen. If you remove them from the can after opening, place them in an air-tight freezer-safe container or bag, and freeze them soon thereafter. These will last at top quality for a couple of months, according to the FDA. Keep in mind the texture of canned sardines will be softer after freezing (and thawing). They will be better suited for cooked dishes like sauces, soups, fish cakes, and casseroles.

Do canned sardines have guts?

Not usually, because the sardines are gutted before they're canned. However, the canneries don't always do an A+ job. You'll rarely, if ever, notice anyway though. It's no concern.

Do you eat the bones in sardines if they have them?

Yes. You can buy sardines that are skinless & boneless. Or, you can buy sardines that come with skin and bones. When the bones are there, they are soft enough to eat them and you should because they're nutritious.

TWO

WHY EAT SARDINES?

If a genie appeared and let me eat any kind of protein, any time I want, simply by snapping my fingers, it would be... a ribeye! (For more, see my book, "The Carnivore Diet Handbook.") But until I find a magic bottle on a beach, I live in the real world of buying groceries and preparing meals for my family, while constantly on the go. In that world, I'm hard pressed to find a more simple and versatile protein solution than sardines!

Sardines are an amazing source of protein for multiple reasons. At a high level, they are:

- Nutrition
- Convenience
- Portability & Travel
- Frugality

I'll address each of these separately, though they intertwine a bit.

Nutritional Benefits of Eating Sardines

I've written a bit already about the nutrition, but it bears repeating. Sardines are one of the most complete foods there are. They're good for your brain, skin, heart, teeth, bones, cells, and to your health in general!

Lose weight, and get lean and strong eating canned sardines. They're high in protein (about 23 grams per can), which is appealing for athletes. High-quality protein provides the amino acids muscles need to repair and rebuild, helping you recover from exercise. Protein is also great for people looking to lose weight because it's satisfying and can keep you from wanting to snack between meals (that is, unless you're snacking on sardines). When you need a quick breakfast, they're so easy to go to instead of cereals or other high carbohydrate foods. By regularly eating animal foods like sardines, you can build a healthy body while losing unwanted fat.

Sardines are high in omega-3 fatty acids EPA and DHA. These vital essential fatty acids decrease inflammation for brain health, heart health, skin health, and joint health. While concentrated fish oil capsules may be a way of obtaining isolated Omega 3 fatty acids, the refining process can eliminate other necessary nutrients that exist in the whole fish, such as Vitamin D, calcium, and the anti-oxidant selenium.

Sardines contain B vitamins (niacin, vitamin B2, vitamin B6, and vitamin B12 - sardines are one of the best sources for B12), and vitamin D (which helps increase absorption of calcium, so they're great for bone health), CoQ 10, selenium, iodine, iron, magnesium, choline, phosphorous (also great for strengthening the bone matrix), calcium (when eating the bones), and potassium.

If you're passionate about longevity, then sardines are for you. They can help prevent dementia and Alzheimer's disease, keep your teeth strong, give you beautiful skin (helps with inflammation, anti-aging, and preventing pimples). They're amazing for your cardiovascular system (they're heart healthy!), and metabolism (the protein and fat are great for this). So, sardines are one of the healthiest foods in the world.

Convenience

Sardines' ultra convenience stems from being canned. Of course, any canned fish or meat is a convenient source of protein, but sardines' low trophic level makes them better than other canned fish (mackerel, etc.) for daily consumption and their nutrient profile and ubiquity make them a much better daily staple than, say, canned ham. Canned sardines offer the following in terms of convenience:

- Portability: Throw a can in your gym bag or suitcase with no chance of making a mess.
- Five-year shelf life
- The long shelf life allows bulk purchasing.
- Bulk purchase and long shelf life means always having some on hand, meaning no planning is required.
- No refrigeration required.
- Ready-to-eat... no cooking necessary.
- Pop-top lids mean you don't need a can opener.
- No dishes required, except a fork (or spoon). Plastic utensils will suffice on the go, as will your fingers, if you don't have any utensils.
- The can is usually aluminum, which is infinitely recyclable, unlike plastic.

You can always have a stash of sardines in your pantry. They're an excellent protein source for preparedness, such as having a 30-day supply on hand for natural disasters or the zombie apocalypse.

Sardine cans pack perfectly in a backpack, duffel bag, or even a purse. They're easy to open with their self-opening tops. The other beauty of them is that, if you don't want to eat them plain, they come prepared and ready to eat with many varieties of sauces. Just pop the top, grab some crackers if you want, and dig in. With other canned fish, like tuna or salmon, "plain" is often your only option.

Eating healthy is a priority for me. As a busy mom, it's not always easy though. Sardines have been life-changing. I can always rely on them to provide superior nutrition. Quality protein in a can. Love it. Pop the top and eat. Very simple. As I wrote before, I've made many meals where I simply cooked pasta or used leftover rice and dumped sardines on top.

Sometimes we have quick blended smoothies made with frozen berries and whole-fat Greek yogurt. On the side, we'll have a can of sardines. My family especially likes this meal combo, because they think it's cool having smoothies for dinner. I think it's cool because it's a nutritious meal with healthy fats and proteins.

Other quick and convenient dinner options include big sandwiches with sardines. For instance, I'll make grilled cheeses with sardines in the middle – freaking AMAZING!!

Or a ham sandwich with mustard, lettuce, sardines, pickles, and a smear of whole-fat Greek yogurt or homemade mayonnaise. Use a quality crusty sourdough bread and add sliced carrots on the side or a cup of soup. It's a fantastic meal!

Portability & Travel

One of my favorite aspects of sardines is that I can easily travel with them, and they're easy to find anywhere in the world. My family is a digital nomad family and we move around the world. Being able to find sardines anywhere we go, so far, is a godsend. I'm relieved to always have some quality animal protein on hand, always easy to find, even in a new city with unfamiliar stores. And, because I don't have to do much in terms of preparation, we can eat them in hotel rooms, in the car, or in a parking lot.

We've taken many road trips where we eat sardines out of the can at gas stations, rest stops, or in shopping mall parking lots. I've taken them to airports and eaten them before boarding a plane. (I'd rather not subject fellow passengers to sardine smell by eating them on a plane.) They're simply a brilliant solution to eating healthy when traveling.

Camping is another no-brainer situation warranting a good stash of sardines. They pack easily in the bottom of any box or bag. They don't require keeping cool in the cooler which is valuable real estate for the food that needs to stay cold. They're nutritionally-turbo charged food packed in a small space!

Frugality

Sardines are the gift that keeps on giving. As if they weren't great enough for their convenience and quality protein, they're pretty cheap, too! Sometimes very cheap.

It's not hard to find sardines for less than a dollar a can. In fact, we've bought cans for under 50 cents in stores all over Europe. As mentioned earlier, warehouse clubs like Costco and Sam's Club carry them, too. Trader Joe's sells sardines as well, though they're not always the smoked variety. That's fine and I like them, it's just a different fish taste, more like a whitefish. Lastly, check out buying them by the carton from Amazon.com, using the super frugal Subscribe-and-Save prices.

The Sardine Habit

So that's a quick rundown of all the great reasons to make sardines a big part of your diet. But what about the taste?

Do sardines taste fishy? It depends on the person. There are ways to ensure they don't (see recipes, chapter 3). My experience eating sardines with different people is that some "beginners" enjoy them most in pâtés, with condiments, or otherwise served in such a way as to make the sardine flavor less strong. However, as people grow to appreciate sardines' awesomeness and badassness, they become accustomed to simply eating them from the can, or perhaps smashed onto some fresh bread. I also know many people who love sardines from the get-go. One of my friends started eating sardines plain, and never looked back. She regularly enjoys the boneless and skinless variety, served plain on crackers.

Sardines as a regular food in your life might seem strange. However, when you eat them in different recipes, you'll enjoy a broad range of flavors and experiences, making them something to look forward to on a regular basis.

Get your family and kids on board with the idea of eating sardines. When it came to enticing my young daughter with sardines, I didn't really give her a choice. I knew they weren't horribly gagging or offensive so it was a pretty safe bet. With a little rewarding she was more willing. Initially, I bribed her with the promise of a nice chocolate treat for eating a sardine. I played up the coolness of the crunchy spine, too. I started with one sardine and, over time, got to the point where she would eat a whole can by herself. She now prefers the can with marinara sauce, or plain if I make them into a sandwich.

For adults in your life who might cringe at the idea of eating sardines, start with the boneless and skinless variety. Use them in a pâté or in a sandwich with condiments, cheese, and maybe bacon. Yum. Strong-flavored condiments such as mustard or hot sauce can do wonders for taming sardines. Same goes for other strong-flavored additions, such as capers or Kalamata olives (see recipes).

Breakfast, Lunch & Dinner

Sardines are great because you can eat them for breakfast, lunch, or dinner.

Breakfast

When I'm in a hurry and don't have time to scramble eggs, I'll wolf down a can of sardines before running out the door. Sardines are great fuel for kids going to school. They're just as easy as eating a bowl of cereal but so much better for your kids' health. If you think kids don't want to eat sardines straight from the can in the morning, or ever, for that matter, don't worry. Whip up one of the pâté recipes in the recipes section, the night before. They'll enjoy that on some toast.

The convenience and speed of being able to quickly eat a can of sardines is brilliant, and cannot be overstated as a serious life pro-tip. On travel days, having cans of sardines on hand is especially helpful because I don't want to dirty any dishes before leaving to catch a plane. Even better is knowing we're fueling up with a great source of protein and nutrients before heading out to a busy day of traveling, especially when your food options might be limited for the rest of the day. For this, be sure to bring some cans along with you!

Lunch

Sardine cans fit into lunches perfectly with their own packaging, if you don't mind eating them straight from the can. All you need is a plastic fork or spoon, but your fingers will suffice in a pinch. If you prefer making the sardines into a recipe, the resulting dish will still pack well, which makes for an easy, delicious, and satisfying lunch. You can keep a stash of cans at work, too. They don't require refrigeration so it's super convenient. Keep a toothbrush and toothpaste at work if you're worried about having sardine smell on your breath.

(Brushing afterward is a good practice regardless of what you eat for lunch, actually.)

Dinner

For dinner, again, sardines are convenient and an easy quality protein to incorporate into any meal. If you get home late from work, you can pop open a can and eat them over rice or pasta or eggs. Or, make a quick salad and eat them with the salad. It's nice to not have to cook the protein for a dinner once in a while (or even more often!).

THREE

RECIPES

For a free, printable .PDF of the recipes in this book, email me at kristen@globalkristen.com.

Beginner Sardine Pâté

Yield 1 to 2 servings

Not so sure about sardines' flavor? Start here! I call this "Beginner Sardine Pâté" because it was the recipe I used most while initially developing my appreciation for the fish. The Kalamata olives, lemon, and mustard are strong enough to make the fish's flavor less noticeable, and enjoy its texture. Over time, you simply dial down the ratio of these ingredients to the sardine, either dialing in your ideal flavor, or working your way toward Sardine Badassness – that is, eating sardines alone.

- 2 cans sardines, packed in water or olive oil, drained
- 2 tablespoons fresh lemon juice
- zest from 1/2 lemon

- 6 Kalamata olives, pitted
- 1 to 2 tablespoons yellow mustard
- 2 tablespoons olive oil
- 2 tablespoons softened butter
- 1 teaspoon freshly chopped rosemary or dill
- Sea salt and freshly ground black pepper, to taste

Using a food processor, fitted with the "s" blade, purée everything until it's a nice smooth texture.

Adjust for salt and lemon.

Eat by the spoon, on crusty bread or crackers, on a salad, with sliced fruit, or with veggies.

Caramelized Onion Sardine Pâté

Yield 1 to 2 servings

This recipe rocks the sardine house. The caramelized onion add a light sweetness along with the honey mustard. Excellent!

- 1 yellow onion, thinly sliced
- 1 to 2 tablespoons butter
- 2 cans sardines, any variety/flavor, drained
- 1 1/2 tablespoons honey mustard
- zest of 1/2 lemon
- 1 tablespoon fresh lemon juice
- 2 tablespoons olive oil
- Sea salt and freshly ground black pepper, to taste

Sauté the sliced onion in the butter over low (or low-medium) heat for 30 minutes, stirring frequently.

Set aside to cool a few minutes.

Place the sautéed onion and remaining ingredients in a food processor, and purée until your desired texture is attained.

Eat by the spoon, on crusty bread or crackers, on a salad, with sliced fruit, or with veggies.

Sardines & Salsa

Yield 1 to 2 servings

A combo that works really well is simply combining sardines and salsa.

- 2 cans sardines, any variety/flavor, drained
- 1/3 to 1/2 jar salsa, to taste
- Squeeze fresh lime juice

Simply smash the sardines and salsa together in a bowl, and squirt on some lime juice.

Enjoy with corn chips, crackers, toast, or by the fork-full.

Relished Sardines

Yield 2 servings

Sardines are relished when served with relish. I love dill pickle relish and bread-and-butter pickle relish – they're both fantastic. Getting that sweet or salty burst of flavor when combined with meaty and oily sardines is so good.

- 2 cans sardines, packed in water, olive oil, or spicy oil
- mustard, any variety, to taste
- scoop of dill pickle relish, bread & butter pickle relish, or sauerkraut
- Freshly ground black pepper, to taste

Put the sardines in a medium sized bowl. Break them up with a fork.

Add the remaining ingredients and mix together.

Eat straight from the bowl, on crackers (or toast), or in a sandwich.

Open-Faced Cracker Sardine Sandwich

Yield 1 serving

Not really a sandwich, but you can do this with bread instead of crackers if you want. A popular way to start with sardines is simply opening the can and putting a little sardine filet on a crunchy cracker. Eat.

- 1 can sardines, any variety/flavor
- Crunchy crackers
- Mustard, optional
- Hot sauce, optional

Open the can of sardines. Get a cracker. Place a sardine filet on the cracker.

Squirt a bit of mustard on it along with a splash of hot sauce.

Enjoy. (Try this with a glass of wine, too!)

Pro Sardine Smash

Yield 2 servings

This is named Pro Sardine Smash because when you become a pro at eating sardines, you don't need all the fancy fixin's or the need to make it into a pâté. Just smash up some sardines, lemon (or lime), add a squirt of mustard. Maybe some hot sauce for good measure. Done.

- 2 cans sardines, any variety/flavor, drained

- Fresh lemon or lime juice, to taste
- Squirt mustard, any variety, to taste
- Hot sauce, optional

Put the sardines in a medium-sized bowl.

Add the remaining ingredients and mash with a fork or spoon.

Eat straight from the bowl, pro.

Dressed Sardines

Yield 1 to 2 servings

This is a way to enjoy sardines dressed in some tasty dressing. This way they're "dressed" up. :)

- 2 cans sardines, packed in water or olive oil, drained
- 2 tablespoons extra virgin olive oil
- Hefty squeeze of fresh lemon juice
- Drizzle of balsamic vinegar
- 1/8 to 1/4 teaspoon freshly minced garlic
- 1 pinch of red pepper flakes
- 1 teaspoon Dijon mustard
- Sea salt and freshly ground black pepper, to taste

Drain the sardines and put them on a plate.

In a small bowl, mix together the remaining ingredients. Pour it over the sardines.

Badass 'n' Plain Sardines

Yield 1 serving

Now, you're ready. You've graduated to loving sardines. You know

they're badass and that you're a badass for eating them this way...
straight from a can. Let's do this!

- 1 to 2 cans sardines, any variety/flavor
- Fork (optional)
- Napkin (optional)

Open the can.

Eat the sardines, and even slurp down the juice (if you're badass
enough).

Wipe the sardine juices that dribbled from your mouth.

Throw away the napkin and can (well, recycle, of course).

Walk away with extra swagger or sass.

Never be stuck without high-quality protein again!

FREE PDF

For a free, printable .PDF of the recipes in this book, email me at kristen@globalkristen.com.

Did you enjoy this book? If so, please leave a review!

As an independent author, your reviews are extremely helpful in getting the word out. After you leave a review, please drop me a line at kristen@globalkristen.com so I can thank you!

Other books by Kristen Suzanne:

The Carnivore Diet Handbook

Recipes with Sardines

Kristen's blog at: GlobalKristen.com

Twitter: @KristensRaw

Instagram: global_kristen